The Easy Water Retention Diet

LINDA LAZARIDES

Other works by Linda Lazarides

Principles of Nutritional Therapy
The Nutritional Health Bible
The Waterfall Diet
Treat Yourself with Nutritional Therapy
The Amino Acid Report
The Big Healthy Soup Diet
Linda's Flat Stomach Secrets
A Textbook of Modern Naturopathy

About the Author

Linda Lazarides is one of Britain's most respected natural health experts, and author of eight titles on health and nutrition. In 1996 she helped the University of Westminster to set up the UK's first degree course in Nutritional Therapy. She is founder of the British Association for Nutritional Therapy, former nutrition editor of the International Journal of Alternative & Complementary Medicine, Founder and Principal of the School of Modern Naturopathy, and for several years worked as a complementary practitioner for the British National Health Service.

©Linda Lazarides 2015
www.naturostudy.org

All rights reserved. This publication may not be transmitted, in any form or by any means, electronic, mechanical, photocopying, recording or otherwise, without the prior permission of the author.

Disclaimer

The information presented herein is not intended as a substitute for medical advice, but every effort has been made to ensure accuracy. The book is sold on the understanding that the publisher and author are not liable for any misconception or misuse of the information provided and shall have neither liability nor responsibility to any person or entity with respect to any loss, damage or injury caused or alleged to be caused directly or indirectly by the said information.

ISBN: 1519191472
ISBN-13: 978-1519191472

DEDICATION

This book is dedicated to the naturopaths, doctors and scientists whose research I have drawn on for my books, especially Australian lymphologist the late Dr. John Casley-Smith

CONTENTS

	Foreword	i
Chapter 1	What is water retention?	1
Chapter 2	How does water retention affect you?	15
Chapter 3	Pregnancy	29
Chapter 4	How do I know if I have water retention?	31
Chapter 5	The causes of type II water retention	36
Chapter 6	The easy water retention diet	55
Chapter 7	Shopping and cooking	58
Chapter 8	Guide to healthy living	69
Chapter 9	Special anti water retention foods	73
App. I	Herbal and nutritional supplements	77
App. II	Recipes	79
App. III	Soy facts	84
	Resources	87

FOREWORD

I would like to thank my readers for their invaluable feedback and support. Dieting to lose water retention does not leave you hungry, but it may require you to change some well-loved food habits and adopt new ones for a few weeks in order to find out which foods are safe for you to eat.

For those of you who find this change a challenge, please continue to read the reviews and encouragements of others, as I do hope you will not give up too soon. Thousands of people with uncomfortable and distressing water retention problems have found relief using the methods described in this book.

CHAPTER ONE
WHAT IS WATER RETENTION?

Water retention is a condition where parts of your body swell up because there is excess water in your blood or in your tissues. The 'tissues' means the fabric of your body, made from tiny units called cells. For instance your body has lung cells, skin, brain and muscle cells. Water can collect in between these cells.

Normally your body maintains the right balance of fluid in your blood and tissues by ensuring that the same of amount of water entering them also leaves them. When you drink a lot of fluid, the water from the fluid is absorbed into your blood. To prevent excessively high water levels in your blood, your kidneys are constantly filtering water out of your blood, turning it into urine and sending it to your bladder so that you can release it by urination.

Your blood vessels—the tiniest ones known as capillaries—also constantly release a watery fluid rich in oxygen and nutrients, through their walls and into your body's tissues. This fluid bathes and nourishes your cells. Once your cells have used up these nutrients, the fluid should be re-absorbed back from your tissues into your blood vessels. So if you suffer from water retention in your tissues, this means that either too much fluid is leaking out of your blood vessels into your tissues, or not enough fluid is returning from your tissues back into your blood vessels.

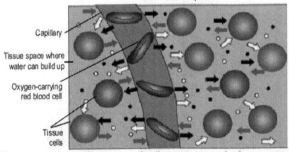

Water leaves the capillary, enters the tissue spaces and releases oxygen and nutrients (black and white arrows) into the cells. Carrying waste products (grey arrows) from the cells, the water then diffuses back into the capillary. Special pores in the capillaries control this process.

There are two types of water retention

Water retention swelling can be in the legs, ankles, knees, feet, tummy, face or fingers, or it can be all over the body. Water retention is also known as fluid retention or oedema (edema). It is a common cause of overweight. If you suffer from water retention, it can be hard to tell whether it is in your blood, or whether your blood is normal and your tissues have too much water.

Water retention in your blood is sometimes known as Type I water retention. It can be serious as it may be a sign of a failing heart and/or kidneys. A possible indicator of water retention in the blood is, if you drink a lot of liquid, instead of urinating a lot more than usual, you swell up instead. If you swell up and also seem to urinate a lot less than you drink, you must consult a doctor. Everyone with water retention should consult a doctor to get their heart and kidneys checked.

Water can also remain in your blood if your kidneys get inflamed. The medical term for kidney inflammation is nephritis. The kidneys can also get inflamed in people with a disease known as lupus. You will see later on that kidney inflammation, even when diagnosed as nephritis, can sometimes be caused by an unusual reaction to eating certain common foods, and can disappear if you carry out a test to avoid these foods.

Most cases of water retention are not serious

If you suffer from water retention but your heart and kidneys have been given a clean bill of health, the excess water may be only in your tissues. Also known as Type II water retention or idiopathic oedema, tissue water retention is a common condition with at least six different causes, including

- Lack of exercise
- Eating the wrong foods

- Not drinking enough water
- Food intolerances
- Vitamin or mineral deficiencies
- Very low calorie diet.

The reason why these are causes of Type II water retention is that they lead to:

- Poor flow in your lymphatic system (which normally helps to drain away excess tissue fluid)
- Imbalances in the hormones which control your sodium levels
- Excessively high sodium levels
- Increased histamine levels
- Weak and leaky blood vessel walls
- In the case of very low calorie diets (or even anorexia nervosa) insufficient protein in your blood.

If you are serious about getting rid of your water retention, it is very important to take your food habits seriously. If you put the wrong kind of oil in a car, or not enough oil, you can maybe drive it for a long time, but it will eventually break down. The human body is the same. The only difference is that we are not born with an instruction manual. Everywhere we look, we see ads for foods that tantalize our taste buds. When we are young, we overindulge in these foods and think nothing of it because everyone around us is doing the same. Most of us don't even know how to cook the kind of foods that keep away water retention and other diseases. Messages like 'Eat Five A Day' are ignored until we get ill. After all, who can be bothered to eat cabbage, carrots and cauliflower every day?

EASY WATER RETENTION DIET

Why drink fresh orange juice when everyone else is drinking sodas or alcohol?

A few people who have healthy eating habits do suffer from Type II water retention, but not many. If you have this problem it is usually because of your eating habits over a long period of time. No matter how normal you think your eating habits are, your metabolism has started to break down because of them, and your water retention will not improve until you start giving your body more of what it really needs, and reducing the foods that stress it most. There's lots of help in this book, so keep reading.

Water retention 'remedies'

Beware of commercial remedies for water retention. Type II water retention is a sign that your metabolism is struggling, and it can't be cured with a pill. Water retention remedies are usually a form of water pills, also known as diuretics, which artificially make your kidneys work harder. They are not effective for Type II water retention, though they are often prescribed by doctors. They will have a temporary effect, but this quickly wears off, and the users soon find they have to take more and more of these pills to avoid the water retention coming back much worse than it ever did before. Here are pleas for help from some of my readers who have taken diuretics for Type II water retention, and regretted it. These stories are sadly very common:

Annie

I guess three years ago my body started to retain water so I started to take a water pill every day. After I started to take them my body got used to them and I couldn't stop taking them. Now they are ruining my life. I'm now taking four pills every day. If I don't take them for one day, my eyes and all my body become big, really big. Especially eye puffiness is really bad. My doctor says I'm healthy apart from my water retention. So I have to stop taking the pills I guess. Tell me please, how long will it take for my body to get healthy again? Will I lose the pounds I've gained because of my water retention? When? When will my eye puffiness be gone? I'm so desperate.

Becca

A few months ago, my weight went from about 115 lbs to fluctuating between 123 and 133 seemingly overnight. I've been from one doctor to another. With each diagnosis, I'm put on meds that have done nothing but make me sick. It seems I have water retention. When I recently went in for an abdominal MRI, I was told I needed a full bladder, so they gave me a whole bottle of water to drink, then another, then another. The wide-eyed radiologist couldn't believe I still couldn't produce any urine, it was hours before I had to use the restroom. After ruling out nearly every major cause or health issue, the general consensus was that the water retention is being caused by my abdominal capillaries leaking, but no one has a clue what to do about it.

EASY WATER RETENTION DIET

I was prescribed two diuretics for the water retention—Dyazide in the morning, Lasix in the evening—but they only seem to be making things worse, so as of yesterday, I stopped taking them. I can tell I'm dehydrated—my skin is dry and itchy, my mouth feels like it's stuffed with cotton, and even my contact lenses are dry and uncomfortable. But I still look like I swallowed a basketball. If I lay on my side, the mass falls to the side like a water balloon. It's plain disgusting—not to mention none of my clothes fit, and I'm always short of breath, congested, head-achy, dizzy, and lethargic.

Natalie

I have had idiopathic edema of my legs and ankles since November of 2009. I am SICK of it. My legs are tingling and tight as I write this and my ankles and feet hurt too. I have been told that I am dehydrated but yet I retain water! Can this be possible? HOW can this be possible? I work at a job where I am walking on a cement floor for 8 hours a day. The ankle/leg with the most swelling has a visible varicose vein with a couple of round red marks (like bruises) on the lower shin. I have taken lasix on and off but the reduction in swelling doesn't last. I am at my wit's end.

Rosa

I have a ridiculous amount of water weight at times 8-10lbs. I am on lasix 160mgs a day. When I first started taking it I was only on 10mg but I have to keep taking higher and higher doses as it stops working. Recently it hasn't been working at all and for the past four days I am still swollen in the feet, ankles, hands and face. I look like I have put on weight. I have had lots of tests to check kidney function, protein, potassium, cbc, everything has come back normal but this problem is getting worse. I need a solution, my doctor wants to take me off the lasix, the dosage is too high and if I try to stop taking it I can't go normally even if I drink a lot of fluid. I really need help.

Robyn

I'm taking oral contraceptives which may be one cause of water retention, and diuretics for my hypertension. I tried to stop the diuretics when my blood pressure stabilized but I got rebound water retention and my BP and water retention shot up again. I didn't weigh so much before I took the diuretics, is there any safe way to get off them?

Suzann

I became physically addicted to diuretics around 18 years ago. I have been taking a combination of lasix and moduretic for this time, and lasix on its own prior to that. I can no longer get any relief unless I take both tablets together. I wish I could stop taking them, but I can't, as when I don't take them I swell up and up and up more every day. Nothing helps, not herbal supplements, nothing. Avoiding salt only helps to stop the rapid rise in weight/swelling, but the swelling and weight gain is simply unbearable. I would give anything to be back to normal, but I can't see how this could ever be possible. I am desperate, feeling this has ruined my life.

Marcie

I have a serious addiction problem with a diurectic called Adco-Retic. It started when I was 25 and I'm now 30 years old and my habit has increased from 1 to 2 to 5 a day and sometimes I take 10 a day depending on my water retention. Please tell me what to do. Can I just stop taking them? I am really wanting to stop but tried before and swelled up so badly that I have just started the bad habit again. Will a kidney cleanse/drinking more water help?

Sadly, Marcie, no it won't help. This is called rebound water retention and is caused by taking diuretics for Type II water retention.

Kate

Wow! What you said is exactly what happened to me. I took a 40 mg Furosemide to relieve bloating and ended up with my skin sore and tender to the touch... all over!! My back and thighs...awful! I was drinking more than usual over the holidays and felt 'puffy'. Big mistake! I think taking the Furosemide made my body do exactly what you described. I feel more bloated and puffy than ever.

Elaine

I have fought this battle with fluid retention for years.

Most every morning my eyes, hands, fingers… are so swollen. I can't wear my jewelry. I take lasix. It helps very little. I only go to the bathroom for a few hours. Then some days I'm not swollen, but I can't figure out why. I ate tomato soup yesterday, and I looked awful and felt awful. I made the soup from tomato juice that I canned. I only put 1 tsp of salt in a quart jar. Then added 1 more when I made the pot of soup. Do tomatoes have that much sodium naturally? Please help me.

Lorelei

I just purchased your book and am very excited to start the diet. I have been struggling with idiopathic edema for 10 years since my son was born. I am up to 160mg of Lasix and 20mg of Prinyvil a day. I have gained over 60lbs in the last 2 years. I drink a ton and I urinate often!! Like 30+ times a day. If I try to stop the meds just for one day, I gain another 10lbs. It is horrible. I have had all kinds of tests. I have never been so miserable in my life. It affects every aspect of my life.

Jeanine

After being on 60mg of frusemide for nearly 8 years, I realized what it was doing to my body. I felt dreadful all the time, and my potassium was really low. I have taken myself off these tablets and seen a doctor, I have also ordered a copy of your book as I am gaining a pound a day in weight which I am sure is fluid. I watch what I eat, so I know that a pound a day is ridiculous. My doctor tells me often it is impossible to get off these tablets. I tell him I am doing it!!!!!

Janis

Dear Linda, I'm a doctor, 33 years old working as a specialist in intensive care medicine and anesthesiology. I suffer from severe water retention. I have tried a lot of different treatments, and have read all the articles in scientific reviews.

My problem started, when I was 20 years old. Around that time I went on a very low-calorie diet (200-500 kcal/day) and lost 11 kilos in four weeks. It was not a healthy diet, sometimes I only ate chocolate. After some time I noticed that before my period I started to get water retention, making my weight rise by 3 to 6 kilos. So I took diuretic tablets from time to time.

My eating habits stayed bad: lot of cakes, chocolate, no fruits and vegetables and very little liquid, because it made me expand. Then my water retention got worse, and was no longer premenstrual but permanent. Four years ago I started trying to control it by taking a diuretic called Amilorid every day.

But still if I spent any time standing, I got water in my abdomen, hands and feet. But at the same time I was dehydrated and constipated. To control the water I reduced my fluid intake to less than 800 ml per day, and I could no longer urinate if I drank more. My medical knowledge told me I had idiopathic oedema. Also, my hands and legs were always cold and sometimes damp.

About 2 month ago I found your diet. In the first 2 weeks on the diet I managed to reduce my diuretic dose by half.

I would like to stop the diuretics completely in order to have a baby with my husband. I don't know what to do, because I can't take diuretics in pregnancy, but I think pregnancy will make the water retention even worse. I'm feeling very sad and hopeless. Dear Linda, please tell me if you think that I will recover if I persevere with this diet. Your scientific work is great, congratulations for it!

Update from Janis 4 months later

There is a great change in my life, I'm pregnant (6 weeks) and still following your diet. I am so much better now, and no longer taking diuretics at all. If I hadn't found your book, I could never have come off the pills, and I would not have been able to have a baby! I'm so very grateful to you.

Why diuretics can make Type II water retention worse

Please be warned. The reason why water pills (diuretics) can be so harmful for Type II water retention is that they dehydrate your blood. Remember that they work by artificially forcing your kidneys to make more urine? That urine is extracted from your blood, and if your blood was normal to begin with, you will quickly become very dehydrated.

Remember too, that in Type II water retention, your water retention is not in your blood but in your tissues. Diuretics are not able to extract water from your tissues - the swollen parts where all the excess water is being retained.

When you take water pills you think you are losing water retention because you pee more, but this water is coming from your blood, not from the waterlogged tissues. Dehydrating your blood is dangerous, so your body learns to hold on to water in order to protect itself. That's why Annie and the others were puffing up so much every time they tried to stop taking the pills.

What if my doctor prescribes diuretics?

We expect our doctor to give us something when we consult him or her. Even though diuretics are only effective for Type I water retention, your doctor doesn't really have anything else to offer, so you are very likely to get a prescription for these pills even if you don't have Type I water retention. My advice is always to ask your doctor this question before leaving: 'If I don't take this medicine, is there any danger to my health?'

If your doctor says 'No' then I recommend you throw away the prescription immediately and start working to repair your metabolism with the methods described in this book. Diuretic medicines are the wrong treatment for all types of tissue (Type II) water retention, whether diagnosed as idiopathic oedema (edema), chronic venous insufficiency or premenstrual water retention. They might appear to work for a while, but before long they will make it worse.

A message from Rita, whose doctor did the right thing

I have had swollen lower legs for the past year. Suprisingly though my actual ankles are skinny, the swelling starts above the ankle bone, I am 5'6" and now weigh about 9 stone 4lbs (130 lbs), not overweight but my normal weight is about 8 stone 7lbs (119 lbs). I also have chubby toes and a pot belly. My doctor said it was pitting oedema and they did a scan on my liver and pelvis in case it was hormones but the results were all fine. Elevating my legs helps but as soon as I stand up the swelling comes back. I hate the appearance of my legs, my stomach is huge and I don't know what to do as my doctor is reluctant to give me water tablets as they put too much strain on the kidneys. Would your diet be suitable for me I have had IBS for the past 5 years and do you think it would help?

Yes Rita, thank God you have a sensible doctor.

If you are taking diuretics and would like to come off them, reduce the dose very, very slowly over a period of several months, in order to minimize the rebound effect.

CHAPTER TWO
HOW DOES WATER RETENTION AFFECT YOU?

Before we discuss the best kind of diet to treat Type II water retention, let's look at the different ways that this problem can affect you. The more you understand about your condition, the easier it will be to commit to what you have to do to get rid of it.

Water weight

One of the most notorious effects of water retention is difficulty with losing weight. If you have been following a weight loss diet for months or even years and just cannot get to a reasonable target weight even if you don't cheat at all, water retention may be the cause.

It is sometimes hard to know if you have water retention or not. Water retention just makes you look fat. It 'pushes out' your normal covering of body fat, making it look much more than it really is. Water is a lot heavier than fat, so water retention gives you a high reading on your weighing scales. When people (including doctors and dieticians) look at you, they assume you are eating too much. All this adds to your belief that you just have too much body fat.

The reason why most weight loss diets, including low-calorie, low-carb and GI diets have little or no effect on water weight, is because they are fat-loss diets. They will help you lose some fat, but then your weight will stick at the same plateau. Take a look at the charts on the next page. They show how, on a low-calorie diet, a typical individual who has both excess fat and water loses weight as calories are reduced to 1,000 kcal per day but then gets stuck at 170 lbs.

Most people like this believe they are still eating too much. In fact 1,000 kcal per day is virtually a starvation diet, and brings risks that you will develop deficiencies of protein, vitamins and minerals. The cause of the plateau is water weight - hidden water which has leaked into the body's tissues and has become stuck there, cooling down the metabolism and adding to the body's bulk and weight.

Water retention cools the metabolism

Weight plateaux have brought thousands of people to the verge of tears. After spending years on 1,000 kcal a day or less, weight can even start to creep upwards again. This is because the body tries to compensate for the lack of food by slowing down its metabolism, making each calorie go

EASY WATER RETENTION DIET

further and last longer. I have known many people who gained weight on only 1,000 Calories a day. Water retention also has its own harmful effect on the metabolism—cooling it down so that fat loss becomes more difficult.

Typical pattern of weight loss when water retention is present

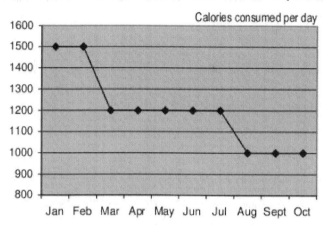

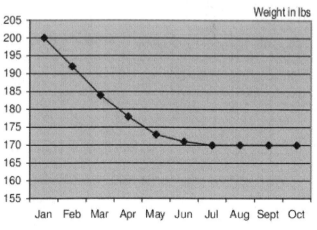

Sometimes hormonal imbalances such as hypothyroidism can have the same effect, but your doctor will usually rule this out with tests. If he or she can find no other reason for your weight plateau, then the possibility of water retention should be considered.

Low-carb diets

A word of caution about low-carb diets. They are ok if you replace sugar and starchy carbs with plenty of fresh fruit and vegetables, and don't eat too much protein and fat. But if you follow the kind of low-carb diet which includes a lot of protein and/or fat, it can have a dehydrating effect on your blood. As you know, dehydration teaches your body to hold on to water, which is not a good thing. All responsible low-carb authors recommend drinking at least eight glasses (two litres) of plain water a day (more in very hot weather or if you are very active), and you should take care to follow this advice to avoid dehydration.

Food allergies and histamine

When starting a low-carb diet, some people have noticed a substantial, almost immediate weight loss accompanied by constant urination. When they come off the diet, they are disappointed to find that all this lost weight is regained straight away. In these cases the individual was probably allergic to wheat, corn or another carbohydrate food. By raising histamine in the body, mild food allergies (not the life-threatening type) are notorious for causing water retention. By following a diet that cuts out the offending food, the water is released and much weight can be lost.

Later in this book I will teach you how to test yourself so that you can identify any particular foods that make you retain water. If your water retention is only brought on by one type of carbohydrate food such as wheat, it does not make sense to avoid all carbohydrate foods like rice and potatoes. There is a special procedure which will help you identify any problem foods.

Fasting

Fasting also bring a few pounds of water loss at the start. The reason is that before you can start to use your body fat as fuel, all your stored carbohydrate must get used up first. This stored carbohydrate (glycogen) is bound with water, and the water is released in the form of urine as the carbohydrate stores disappear. You may appear to be a couple of pounds lighter after fasting for 24 hours, but this isn't real weight loss. The weight will return as soon as you begin to eat again.

By following the diet given later in this book, thousands of people have managed to lose stubborn pounds of water weight which they had been trying to shift for years.

Swollen tummy

Many women suffer from water retention before their period. Known as premenstrual water retention, this can cause a very swollen, uncomfortable tummy. The reason for the swelling is a hormonal imbalance which makes the body retain sodium. The correct balance of sodium in the body is maintained not just by consuming water, but also by a complex interplay of different hormones including anti-diuretic hormone (ADH) and dopamine. If a woman is not properly nourished with foods that provide the right vitamins and minerals, then when her hormones change pre-menstrually, it can affect her sodium balance.

Another cause of a swollen tummy was mentioned in one of the case reports earlier in this book. In this case, water was leaking from the small blood vessels in the woman's tummy and collecting in her abdominal cavity. She could actually feel it sloshing around.

This type of tummy swelling is not related to female hormones but to the strength of the walls of the smallest blood vessels in the body. If these vessels are not properly nourished, they can leak fluid, either into the tissues, or, in this case, into the space between the tummy's internal organs.

In the diet section of this book we will look at the foods which you need to eat to keep your small blood vessels strong and healthy so that they don't leak excessive amounts of fluid.

You can also develop a swollen tummy if you have been following a very low-calorie diet for a long time. Very low-calorie diets may provide so little food that you become deficient in protein. But sufficient protein is needed to keep fluid in your blood, and prevent excessive amounts of fluid leaking into your tissues and into your abdominal cavity, where it causes bloating. This kind of tummy swelling is exactly the same as seen in pictures of starving people in developing countries. Yours may not be so noticeable. You might just think you are a bit fat in that part of your body.

Here is a story from my case-book.

Paula

Paula was only 22, and had recently started a new job after leaving university. Her mother brought her to see me because she was very worried. Paula had been trying to control her weight by yo-yo dieting since she was 13. At first the weight came off easily but Paula could not stay off the chocolates and sweets (candies) so she quickly put it back on again. Each time she put on more weight than she had previously lost. When she was 18 Paula became a vegan—a strict vegetarian who eats no animal or fish produce at all, including dairy products and eggs. This was because she felt this way of eating was kinder to animals, which she loved.

Unfortunately her vegan diet did not help Paula lose weight. By age 20, Paula was desperate. Her metabolism seemed to have slowed down to a halt. She ate almost nothing at all. Breakfast consisted of black coffee, lunch was green salad leaves without dressing, and dinner was steamed vegetables and a thin rye cracker. Paula was most of all concerned about her tummy, which was quite large. She also thought the rest of her body was fat too, though to me it looked more like water retention than fat, which does not look rounded but tends to hang in folds.

I asked Paula if she would consider eating yoghurt to

boost her protein intake. I said that I thought she was suffering from protein deficiency and that this was slowing down her metabolism and giving her water retention, especially in her tummy.

Paula said she would think about eating more protein, but was not keen on the idea. She was really fixated on eating as few calories as possible. Like many people who have been unsuccessfully trying to control their weight for years, she had become a little obsessed by the calories=overweight connection. I found it hard to gain her trust, and after she did not return to see me again for some months, I thought that she was probably continuing in her old ways. I was pleasantly surprised when she appeared again six months later and reported that she had lost 10 pounds by eating more protein.

Because they think they are fat, people with water retention often go on a very low-calorie diet of 1,000 calories a day or less, believing this is the only way to lose weight. Unfortunately a very low-calorie diet is more likely to worsen water retention and aggravate your weight problem. Here is a message from one of my readers.

Tessa

I gain 6 inches of fluid around my ankles and 12 inches daily around my waist and I am on 5 different diuretic medications daily. I am retaining more than 70 lbs of fluid. What can I do and why could this be? My doctor just keeps putting me on more meds and they are not helping I only eat 1100 cals a day.

EASY WATER RETENTION DIET

Anorexia and bulimia of course involve a very low calorie intake, and people with these problems may also not eat enough protein to avoid developing water retention. Here are some messages from my readers.

Pat

I've been bulimic for 20 years, and my weight has been up and down, also my electrolytes. E.g. potassium has been as low as 1.6. My periods stop and start. My problem now is massive swings in water retention. I can't function as I feel so bloated. I am still vomiting on a regular basis.

Eric

I have a stomach problem. I think it's due to my bulimia. My stomach gets like bloated and in the front part of my stomach I have like some stuck fluid and it's just sitting there.

Swollen legs, feet, ankles

If your heart and kidneys are ok and you are not a pregnant woman, then your swollen legs, feet and ankles have probably been diagnosed as 'chronic venous insufficiency' or CVI, which simply means 'weak leg veins'. This is a condition mostly found in older people, and is often accompanied by varicose veins. Varicose veins are those discoloured, bulging, knotted veins which can be seen in some older people, and can become very inflamed and painful.

In people with CVI, the valves in the leg veins are too weak, and blood which is trying to travel up your legs to your heart keeps slipping down again. This increases the pressure in all your tiny leg veins and capillaries, and forces fluid out of their walls and into the tissues, where it collects and causes swelling. Movement and exercise helps with the blood flow in your legs, so standing or sitting still can really aggravate this problem. Hot weather also tends to aggravate swollen legs, as the veins expand with heat and become even more leaky.

In the diet section of this book you will find lists of foods that help to keep blood vessels strong, and herbal medicines that can speed up the repair process and help get the blood flowing in your legs.

Long distance flights can also cause swollen legs, feet and ankles. This is due to a combination of pressurized cabins and many hours of sitting completely still. If someone has latent idiopathic oedema, a long-distance flight can suddenly trigger a severe gain in water weight, which remains after the flight and will not go away on its own. Here are two messages from my readers:

Jonathan

I am a 40 yr old male. I have recently changed my lifestyle for quite a healthy one and have been losing about 1kg per week for the last 10 weeks. I normally weigh myself once a week and was stunned to find that I actually weigh 1kg more than a week ago just after getting back from a 2-day business trip. I have not over-indulged and even went for a run while I was away. Can it be possible that I retained water from the 6 hours drive there and back and from sitting in a meeting for 2 straight days?

Salwa

I am a patient diagnosed with idiopathic oedema. I am also a doctor (gynaecologist).

My water retention started suddenly during an 18-hour flight from Canada to the Middle East in 2001. I had been under stress due to the completion of my residency program and having my Royal College exams and American Board exam. During this flight I gained an incredible 7 kilos. Even after resting for two weeks after the flight, this water retention did not subside at all.

When I found the problem would not go away, I underwent very thorough medical testing, including echocardiography, MRI and all metabolic tests and hormones. All tests were normal yet in spite of this I was retaining water in all my tissues, including lungs and abdomen. I even went to the Mayo clinic in the USA to try to get help, but my water retention only got worse and worse. Five weeks ago I started to develop a new symptom—a constant feeling of needing to empty my bowels. An endoscopy revealed I now had water retention in my bowel wall.

Four weeks ago I found a copy of your book the Waterfall Diet with a newspaper seller as he was cleaning his booth. I read it and hoped it might work so I started it straight away. I got a lot of pain in the first few days of the diet, but I soon started to feel a lot better. I am keen to come and consult you in the UK.

So far in only four weeks I have already lost 4-6 kilos on your diet, depending what time of day I weigh myself. Before the diet, I had severe abdominal pain with harrying diarrhoea and a constant feeling of needing to empty my bowels. These feelings are almost gone. I also had pain and burning sensations in the soles of my feet and these too have almost gone. The regular headaches I used to suffer from have completely gone, and if I sometimes get one now, it is very mild and I don't need to take painkillers. I feel great and I'm much lighter and more energetic.

Slow metabolism

Water retention increases the distance between blood vessels and cells in your body, and expands the tissue space between cells. It dilutes nutrients and oxygen, and damages cell-to-cell communication. Cell membranes become more permeable to toxins which they would not normally absorb. One of the effects of this waterlogging is to slow down your metabolism, making it much harder for you to burn off your calories. People with water retention find that normal weight loss diets just don't work, or else they work up to a point, but the last 20 pounds or so just will not shift.

Before you can boost your metabolism, you need to get rid of the water retention. Here is another story from my

EASY WATER RETENTION DIET

casebook:

Georgie, age 49, worked in a care home for people with Alzheimer's disease. She was eating as little as she could, and got plenty of exercise, being on her feet most days from 7 am until sometimes 9 pm, up and down stairs. But no matter how hard she tried, her weight would not budge from 12 stone (168 lbs). Worst of all, it was creeping slowly upwards although for the last four years she was eating little but salad with a small portion of lean grilled meat or fish, and thin wheat crackers.

I wondered if Georgie suffered from hidden water retention, so I asked if any parts of her body felt swollen. She had not noticed any swellings, except for her knees. Georgie's doctor had diagnosed her with osteoarthritis because her knees were painful and swollen, made much worse by walking upstairs. Marjorie had to take painkillers every day for her knee pains.

There was such a lot of swelling around both Georgie's knees that it didn't really make sense unless it was related to a more general body water retention problem. I told Georgie that I believed she suffered from hidden water retention in other parts of her body, and that there was only one way to find out - to try my water retention diet (also known as the Waterfall Diet) on an experimental basis.

Georgie was keen to try anything if it could help her lose weight, and started the diet immediately. After a few days, I got an excited phone call. 'I think I've been suffering from water retention all these years' she said. 'I've been peeing it all away - several gallons so far. My clothes are so loose they're hanging off me!'

Georgie peed so much that she weighed 15 lbs less by the end of the first week on my diet. The peeing and weight loss stopped for a few days, and then started again. Two weeks later when she saw me again, she was ecstatic. 'I've been constantly on the loo again and have lost another 7 lbs. My knee swelling has disappeared, the pains have completely gone, I no longer need painkillers, and I'm feeling so full of energy for the first time in years that I'm going to start an exercise class!'

Georgie lost a total of 22 lbs of water retention, and as long as she didn't eat the wrong foods, it never came back again. Within a few short months she was looking 10 years younger. After getting rid of the excess water, Georgie's metabolism had improved so much that she also managed to lose a few pounds of body fat – something that was not possible while her body was waterlogged. Georgie was my most successful case ever.

Sadly, so many doctors won't believe people when they say they have been working hard at dieting. Some will more or less accuse you of stuffing yourself with chocolate bars and just not admitting it. I have known people driven to the verge of tears because they were already on a starvation diet, but instead of getting slimmer they were getting fatter.

Don't be one of these people. The diet in this book may be the answer for you, so don't lose hope.

CHAPTER THREE
PREGNANCY

Water retention is very common in the later stages of pregnancy, and causes swollen legs and ankles. During pregnancy, levels increase of several hormones, such as cortisol, oestrogens, and progesterone. These hormonal changes alone can promote water retention, especially if your body already has a tendency to this problem, but there are other causes too. Swelling in the legs, ankles and feet is mostly caused by the weight of the baby pressing down on a large vein in your pelvis. This vein is called the vena cava, and carries blood from your lower body back to your heart. Pressure on this vein makes blood flow more slowly so that it pools in your legs and ankles. The extra pressure in your legs forces the smallest veins to leak fluid into the tissues of your legs. Warm weather, and spending too much time on your feet aggravates the problem.

The most important tip to help control this problem is

to lie on your left side, which helps to relieve the pressure on the vena cava.

The hormonal changes of pregnancy, combined with the unborn baby's extra nutritional demands, can also trigger water retention in a more serious way, which has the very undesirable effect of raising the mother's blood pressure. High blood pressure in pregnancy is known as pre-eclampsia, and must be controlled for the sake of both mother and baby. Here is a story from my case-book.

Heather

Heather's mother brought her to see me in 1992 when Heather was seven months pregnant. It was her first pregnancy. She was 23 year old and a vegetarian.

Heather had been diagnosed with both severe anaemia and high blood pressure. Her doctor had prescribed iron supplements for the anaemia, but Heather's anaemia just kept getting worse, so he wanted to keep her in hospital to give her iron injections. Heather didn't want this at all.

The hospital dietician had given Heather a list of foods to eat to improve her anaemia, but Heather had a real problem with eating. She had almost no appetite at all. She did not suffer from anorexia nervosa, but she just could not eat. While the rest of the family had a complete meal, Heather might pick only at a piece of cheesecake. Yet in spite of this she was very overweight, which of course was because she was retaining a lot of water.

By the time she consulted me, Heather's skin was extremely pale, and her legs were severely swollen. Both

EASY WATER RETENTION DIET

Heather and the baby were at risk due to her sky-high blood pressure and serious anaemia.

I asked about Heather's diet history, and unfortunately it was problematic, with a lot of fried and convenience food, white bread, chocolate, and biscuits (cookies). When I analysed all of Heather's small symptoms, I found that she also suffered from permanent sores in her mouth and for the first few months of her pregnancy she had felt nauseous 24 hours a day.

To a naturopathic nutritionist, these symptoms were very significant, and it became clear to me that Heather's anaemia was being caused, not by an iron deficiency, but by a completely different mineral—zinc. People with a severe zinc deficiency have no appetite, and their sores do not heal well. The more iron Heather took for her anaemia, the worse her zinc deficiency was bound to get, as iron competes with zinc for absorption by the body. A zinc deficiency is also dangerous in pregnancy as zinc is needed for growth, so the baby's development could be impaired.

I asked Heather to obtain permission from her doctor to stop the iron supplements, and I gave her a some zinc supplements and some instructions to help control her water retention.

To her doctor's amazement, Heather's haemoglobin levels started to rise within days, her blood pressure went down, and she went on to produce a healthy baby.

My water retention diet is safe for use in pregnancy, and can not only help to prevent swollen legs and ankles, but can also help to control blood pressure.

CHAPTER FOUR
HOW DO I KNOW IF I HAVE WATER RETENTION?

If you can answer yes to any of the questions below, there is a strong possibility that you may have water retention.

- Have you worked hard to lose weight using conventional methods, and found that you cannot get below a certain weight even if you persevere for months or years?
- Press a fingernail firmly into your thumb-pad. Does it stay deeply dented for more than a second or two?
- Press the tip of your finger into the inside of your shin-bone. Can your finger make a dent?
- Water retention often collects in the legs and ankles. Do your ankles ever swell up?
- Does your shoe size seem to increase as you get older?
- Do your rings sometimes seem not to fit you any more?

EASY WATER RETENTION DIET

- Do you get a major swelling problem in hot weather?
- Water retention can cause bloating. Is your tummy often tight and swollen?
- If you are a woman, do you often suffer from breast tenderness?
- If you are a woman, do you gain weight pre-menstrually?
- Does your weight ever fluctuate by several pounds within the space of only 24 hours?

What is causing my water retention?

We will assume you have Type II water retention (all cases of water retention need to be checked out by a doctor just in case you have the more dangerous Type I). This book is not suitable for people with Type I—you should follow your doctor's advice.

Answer the following questions to see which causes of Type II water retention might apply to you

Section A

1. Are you a female with water retention mostly in the form of tummy bloating and/or breast tenderness?
2. Is your water retention mostly in your legs and ankles?
3. Does your water retention seem to be all over, with puffiness in many parts of your body?
4. Do you also suffer from regular headaches, skin rashes, sinus congestion or irritable bowel?

Section B (score 1 for each yes answer)

1. Do you mostly eat convenience food and deep-fried food?
2. Do you mostly drink sodas, tea, coffee or alcohol?
3. Do you eat or drink sugary items more than twice a day?
4. Are you on a very low-calorie diet to control your weight?

Answers

A1 with a B score of 1 or more

You probably have vitamin and mineral deficiencies which are disrupting your hormones. (Pregnancy can also cause swollen legs, due to the weight of the baby on your pelvic veins.)

A1 plus B4

Very low calorie diets can cause deficiencies of vitamins, minerals and protein, all of which can cause water retention, especially in the tummy area.

A2 with a B score of 1 or more

You may be lacking in the nutrients found in fresh fruit and vegetables, and this may be weakening the veins in your legs.

A3 or A4

If you have a high B score, it looks like you have a few dietary habits that need to be improved before you will be able to make a difference to your water retention. You may also have developed an intolerance to certain foods, causing you to make too much histamine.

CHAPTER FIVE
THE CAUSES OF TYPE II WATER RETENTION

Now that you have some idea of what may be causing your water retention, here are some explanations of how these causes lead to the symptoms of water retention. The reason why these explanations are important is that to be really effective, my water retention diet (Waterfall Diet) has to be done strictly. It is not like ordinary weight loss diets, where you may be allowed 'a little of what you fancy'. It is a diet to relieve a medical condition.

Water retention cause number 1
Vitamin and mineral deficiencies

Vitamin and mineral deficiencies in the western world are much more common than we think. The problem is that most of us eat quite large amounts of foods which have had most of their vitamins and minerals removed, for example:

- White flour, white pasta, white bread etc.
- White rice
- Sugar (both brown and white), as found in candy, cookies, chocolate and confectionery, ice-cream, desserts and soft drinks.
- Refined vegetable oils
- Fats in desserts, bakery and patisserie products, ice cream, potato chips and crisps, mayonnaise, dips, deep-fried foods and peanut butter, etc.

If 50 per cent or more of the calories you eat come from these foods, then you are only getting 50 per cent of the vitamins and minerals that you could be getting from a more natural diet.

Water retention is only one of the potential results of vitamin and mineral deficiencies. They can also cause skin rashes or spots, fatigue, insomnia, split or brittle fingernails, mood swings, palpitations, PMS or nervous problems. Here is a story from my case-book.

Emma

Emma was 25 and was studying beauty therapy. Her boyfriend brought her to consult me because she was always tired. She went to college most days on the bus, but although the bus stop was only 200 yards from her house, she was exhausted by walking this short distance. Because of the lack of exercise, Emma was putting on weight and she also had a lot of premenstrual symptoms: bloating, breast tenderness and temper tantrums.

When I asked Emma what she ate for her meals, she

confessed that she didn't know how to cook, so she never cooked anything. Breakfast was cereal, and sometimes dinner was cereal too. Lunch was a sandwich and a packet of potato crisps. The only time Emma ever had a proper cooked meal was when she went to her mum's house once every two weeks or so.

It was clear to me that Emma was suffering from premenstrual water retention due to multiple vitamin and mineral deficiencies. Her skin was bad too, and for a beautician that was not a good advertisement. Insomnia left dark circles under Emma's eyes, which added to the problem.

The first thing was to get Emma eating some fresh food, so I gave her a recipe for an easy home-made vegetable soup, and her boyfriend helped her with the shopping. Emma put potatoes, onions, tomatoes, carrots and shreds of green cabbage in the soup, and added olive oil, a stock cube and some herbs to make it taste good. I also asked her to change her breakfast cereal to unsweetened cornflakes, which are much more nourishing than the very sugary product she had been buying. She agreed to take a multivitamin and mineral product to help speed up her recovery from the effects of her nutritional deficiencies.

Luckily as Emma was young, she responded very quickly to these measures, and within only two weeks her energy levels had improved enormously. Her premenstrual symptoms improved by about 50 per cent within a month, and by three months she hardly noticed any premenstrual symptoms at all.

EASY WATER RETENTION DIET

Even if you feel you can live with your water retention, and feel it is preferable to making changes in your diet or lifestyle, you do need to be aware that vitamin and mineral deficiencies can in time lead to more serious problems too. Take a look at some of the older members of your family who have the same dietary habits as you. Do they have any health problems? When you look at them, you may be looking at yourself a few years down the line. A lot of the health problems which have been attributed to inherited 'genetic' factors can also be due to inheriting dietary habits. If you can start to develop more healthy habits you may be able to prevent not just water retention, but other problems too.

Several nutrients are especially important to maintain a healthy water balance:

- Vitamin B6
- Magnesium
- Iron
- Selenium
- Flavonoids (from fruit and vegetables and their skins)

Vitamin B6

This is mostly found in bread made from whole-meal flour, wheatgerm, pumpernickel bread, brown rice, oats, nuts, sunflower and sesame seeds, avocado pears and bananas. If you don't eat some of these foods every day, you could be at risk of deficiency. Vitamin B6 is inactivated by alcohol, the contraceptive pill and hormone-replacement therapy. I come across people with vitamin B6 deficiency all the time. Unlike calcium, iron and vitamins B1, B2 and B3, it is not artificially added to white flour to help put back some of the nutrients that are lost when flour goes through the refining process.

A vitamin B6 deficiency leads to higher levels of hormones which slow down water excretion. In women this is often worse pre-menstrually, and causes tummy bloating and swelling. Vitamin B6 is also needed for your body to use zinc, a mineral that plays a vital role in immunity.

Magnesium

While playing just as important a role as calcium in the body, magnesium is not artificially added to white flour, so you have to get it from foods like whole-meal bread, pumpernickel, brown rice, oats, nuts, sunflower and sesame seeds, cocoa powder, soybeans and leafy green vegetables. If you neglect to eat a variety of these foods every day you could be playing Russian Roulette with your body's water balance. Coffee is an enemy of magnesium, as it makes you excrete magnesium in your urine.

If you don't get enough magnesium, your body will suffer from these problems which can lead to water retention:

- Reduced potassium levels
- Sodium accumulation
- Increased levels of aldosterone, a hormone which slows down your kidneys.

EASY WATER RETENTION DIET

The high blood pressure (known as pre-eclampsia) which can occur in pregnancy, is due to low magnesium levels causing water retention. Extra water in your tissues tends to raise your blood pressure, and the extra nutritional demands of pregnancy can aggravate a borderline magnesium deficiency.

Iron

Most people know that a lack of iron leads to anaemia (anemia). Anaemia causes oxygen starvation and an overworked heart. In time a severe anaemia problem can lead to Type I water retention.

A lack of zinc, vitamins B6 or B12 or folic acid can also cause anaemia. Iron deficiency also reduces the efficiency of your thyroid gland, which governs your metabolism.

Selenium

There are several countries in the world, including the UK and New Zealand, where selenium levels in the soil are extremely low, and people in these countries do not get enough selenium in their diet. Selenium is particularly important for your kidneys, and researchers have found that people with a selenium deficiency have less efficient kidneys. Since your kidneys remove excess fluid from your body and so help to avoid water retention, it is important to look after them. Fish, seafood and Brazil nuts are the best sources of selenium in these countries.

Flavonoids

Flavonoids are pigments found in fruits and vegetables. The purple pigment found in blueberries, bilberries, blackberries and black cherries, are the most important flavonoids to help keep your tiny blood vessels strong so that they don't leak too much fluid into your tissues.

My water retention diet later in this book aims to help your body replace its missing nutrients so that it can start to repair your water retention problem, and hopefully also any other ailments which may have been developing at the same time.

Water retention cause number 2
The salt connection

Some people suffer from water retention because they consume too much salt, salty foods or other sodium-rich foods such as baking powder or certain additives like MSG found in processed foods. Sodium forms part of salt (its chemical name is sodium chloride) and is the part of the salt molecule that makes you retain water. The reason is that when sodium levels are high, the body will always try to dilute them. That is why salty foods make you thirsty. Your body makes you thirsty so that you will drink water to dilute the sodium. It will then hold on to the water until it gets the chance to excrete the sodium.

Dehydration also stimulates the body to retain sodium. That is one reason why we are recommended to drink plenty of water every day. Tea, coffee, and especially alcohol, have a strong diuretic effect, and will dehydrate you if you don't make up for the lost fluid by drinking sufficient water. Alcohol actually switches off the safety mechanism which reduces urine production when you are dehydrated. This can be quite dangerous as you will continue losing fluid and getting more and more dehydrated. Sugary drinks can also promote water retention. They make you retain sodium by stimulating your body to produce more insulin.

Here is a story from my case-book.

Jamie

Jamie, aged 32, loved salt. He put extra helpings of salt on food that was already well-seasoned, and his favourite foods were salami, smoked fish and salted nuts—all high-sodium foods. Jamie consulted me for a weight loss problem and also for the pains in his joints. His fingers were especially painful, but he had swollen knees and ankles too.

As Jamie's high sodium intake was the obvious thing to work on, to help reduce his water retention, I aimed at that first, and counselled him to avoid all forms of salt and salted food for a week. Processed and convenience foods like bread and canned food tend to contain quite a lot of hidden salt, so I advised Jamie to read all labels carefully and try to eat only food that he had prepared himself for the next week.

Over the next week, Jamie lost an incredible 5 lbs of water retention, and the pain and swelling in his fingers disappeared. It turned out that he was really sensitive to sodium, and was able to tolerate eating much less salt than other people. Eating even a small amount of salt made Jamie retain so much water in his joints that they became swollen and painful.

In an indirect way, sugar can also make your sodium levels rise. Your body produces a hormone called insulin when you eat sugary foods and drinks. Research from the University Hospital of South Manchester in England shows that high levels of insulin not only slow down your excretion of sodium, but are also detrimental to your kidneys, your vital water release organ.

Water retention cause number 3
Histamine (food allergies)

Some people get water retention because eating a particular food makes their body produce too much histamine. Histamine makes your small blood vessels leaky, so that more fluid escapes into your tissues. It can also affect the functioning of your kidneys. Histamine-related water retention can be the most severe kind of Type II water retention, but it is also lost the most quickly – by avoiding the food or foods that trigger it.

If your water retention is histamine-related, you may find that you suffer from one or more of the symptoms below. If you do, this is a sure sign that you will get great benefits from following the diet advice in this book.

- Regular headaches or migraine
- Fingers or knees regularly puffy or painful

EASY WATER RETENTION DIET

- Chronic catarrh or congestion of nose or sinuses
- Asthma or hay fever
- Bloating and flatulence after eating
- Frequent diarrhoea or irritable bowel
- Eczema or other skin rashes

Researchers at the Henri Mondor Hospital in Créteil, France, have observed that some people's kidneys become so inflamed from eating certain foods that they stop working. Severe water retention then accumulates. The researchers found that the problem foods vary from person to person, but that once they are identified and withdrawn from the patient's diet, the kidneys work normally again and the water is rapidly shed by urination over the next few weeks. This is surely the closest thing to instant weight loss!

Why does a food make your body create histamine?

There are a number of theories, but the most likely is that the intestines get irritated by bacterial imbalances, and become mildly inflamed. When this happens, food particles that the body hasn't properly digested get absorbed from the intestines into the blood, where antibodies react with them, producing histamine. A vicious circle tends to develop and the only way it can be stopped is to find out what the problem food is and stop eating it for a while. A food that you were previously able to eat with no problems can start to trigger water retention in this way.

Allergy to a food or a food additive can also cause sudden swellings, as experienced by Steven, who sent me this message:

For a year and a half I've been sitting in the law library most days for long periods of time. My diet is not the best: McDonalds, Chinese, fish, veggies, cup of noodles, snacks at the vending machine and sodas. One day I had two cup of soup while studying at the library and my toes and then my legs began to swell. In 10 minutes they swelled up so bad that my skin split open.

Water retention cause number 4
Toxins

Our bodies are exposed to toxins all the time, from airborne pollutants to pesticides and bacterial toxins absorbed from our intestines. Inflammation is the body's attempt to get rid of toxins, and is likely to occur wherever toxins are stored in our body. Inflammation tends to generate swelling and water retention.

There are many things we can do to help the body break down and eliminate toxins. Our liver especially needs B vitamins, protein and antioxidants. Certain herbs and spices—for instance milk thistle and turmeric—can give it much-needed support. Vegetables in the cruciferous family (broccoli, cabbage and brussels sprouts) are especially helpful to the liver as they help to create enzymes which break down toxins.

A number of prescription drugs and over-the-counter medicines are treated by the body as toxins, and are notorious for promoting water retention. Some of the main categories include:

- Beta-blockers
- Calcium-channel blockers
- Clonidine
- Methyldopa
- Insulin
- Metoclopramide
- Oral contraceptives and HRT/ERT drugs
- Steroids
- Some NSAIDs (non-steroidal anti-inflammatory drugs)
- Danazol

You may not recognize these names as they are 'generic' names, not brand names. If you are not sure what you are taking, try searching on the Internet to find out if your medication falls into one of these categories.

Here are some messages from my readers, who discovered that they developed water retention soon after treatments with prescription drugs.

Lonnie

I'm in remission for breast cancer and had my last chemo in September. I am gaining weight like crazy. The water in my legs is bad. I get big bumps like boils and water comes out when I squeeze them. My legs stay indented for quite a while. I'm on 40mg lasix once daily. What causes the bumps? Sometimes they are behind my knee or around my ankle.

Jodie

I started to take diet pills (dyromine) about 5 weeks ago and in the first week I put on 3.8kg. By the end of the 4th week I had put on 5kg. I have now stopped the diet pills as I thought that maybe I'm having a problem with fluid retention. I went to my doctor but he just told me that some diet pills don't agree with everyone. This has caused me great distress. My son is 3 years old and some people think that I am having another child since a lot of the time my stomach looks like I am 4 months pregnant.

Dorothy

I have swelling in my knees, legs, and feet, ever since I had a complete knee replacement done. I am on methadone for the pain in my back and knees and feel that this might be the culprit of my problems. I need to find a natural way to get the pain to go away. I don't have time to sit around with my feet up at all times. I hardly eat anymore and I just feel like I am gaining weight no matter what.

Betty

I have been experiencing a lot of hormonal imbalances and I was given the Pill to balance them (took it for 1 year and a half). However, the pill filled me up with water and even gave me lots of mental problems so I decided to stop it (like 8 months ago). Now that I stopped the pill my hormones still are not balanced though some of the water has drained.

EASY WATER RETENTION DIET

Francis

Been taking Tramadol for pain and now my legs and ankles are swollen. Could it be from the medication?

Twana

I'm taking the depo provera birth control pill. I have gained a lot of weight. My fingers and feet swell early in the morning or after work in the evening. Also I get a cold burning feeling in my feet at times. I feel really tired, moody and nervous all the time.

Tania

I suffered severe edema when I was pregnant with my daughter (6 years ago). Within a month of getting pregnant I had gained 3 stone (42 lbs), I went from skinny to what my obstetrician described as obese. My midwife said it was normal weight gain even though I went up at least 8-10 dress sizes. My skin just ripped to pieces, I was in agony and my skin was so itchy I cried constantly and felt like I wanted to cut my legs off just to stop the pain. I couldn't even bath my daughter or change her for 2 months as my whole body was so swollen. Luckily my mum is amazing and did all of this for me.

A similar thing happened when I had a mirena coil fitted. After 24 hours I was so swollen I ended up in A&E, screaming in pain and begging someone to remove it. I have spent £18,000 on reconstructive surgery just to get rid of the excess skin caused by the oedema, I even had liposuction thinking maybe I was fat. But the majority of the lipo loss was fluid.

I'm now vegan, no longer drink alcohol, never use salt and have stopped taking the pill as I think the hormones may be doing more harm than good. I've been taking butchers broom, uva ursi, cornsilk, magnesium and potassium supplements as your book suggested that these may help.

Tonight I have been to see my doctor. He told me that I will have this condition for life, and if I get pregnant again the same thing will happen and my body will be unable to cope, I asked him about diet and he said that this will make no difference. You are my final hope, is there anything else that I can do?

Lauren

My water retention started 3 yrs ago with injections for varicose veins in my legs. After about 4 sessions over several months, I started retaining water, up to 5 lbs by 3 in the afternoon. It subsides at night and doesn't respond to reducing my salt consumption. No help from several Drs. Lymphatic massages get rid of it temporarily. My diet is organic, rotation and I have added in several foods from an elimination diet. The water is throughout my body, accumulates daily, being tiring and uncomfortable. I am 5'8", 113lbs and exercise daily hoping to help circulation and move fluid. I am 49, on bio identicals for hormones, compound T3 and T4 for thyroid.

EASY WATER RETENTION DIET

Marcus

I am on Lexapro for panic disorder and have gained 10 lbs.

Amanda

When I have more than 1g of sodium a day I gain so much weight. I have to avoid sodium and eat many bananas till it goes away but now and then it comes back. It started after I took a tablet called chantix which I took for 8 weeks and it has really messed me up somehow.

Hope

Since I used chantix to stop smoking, I cannot eat salt, MSG, baking powder etc. without having instant weight gain. I weigh myself each night to check, and if I have gained loads of lbs then I make sure I eat foods with zero salt, but its taking weeks for my weight to go back to normal. Cutting salt to zero just isn't working, I don't know what else I can do.

Marie

I have swelling of the feet, legs, hands and abdomen. I also have trouble breathing. I have gained 12 pounds in two weeks and cannot walk more than a few feet or lay down flat without having trouble breathing. Would water pills help this condition? About the same time this all began to happen my doctor changed my blood pressure medicine and told me to take 1/2 tablet twice a day of a beta-blocker called labetalol.

Teresa

Nearly 50 years ago, at age 19 I went on a birth control pill that was very strong. I quickly developed fluid retention in lower legs and ankles. Even when I came off the pill a few years later, the fluid retention didn't clear up, and I still have it. For the past 20 years I've had high blood pressure, currently under control with a small dose of Atenolol (12.5mg) and Amlodipine (2.5mg). I understand that this type of medication can cause water retention, but then I had it anyway, and wouldn't say it's any worse for being on these meds. I'm not overweight and am not conscious of fluid anywhere else in the body. Do you think your diet would help me? I already eat very healthily, loads of veg and salad, fairly low carbs, more than adequate protein.

Water retention cause number 5
Dehydration

Did you know that by the time you feel thirsty, you are already at least 2 per cent dehydrated? Dehydration teaches your body to hold on to water, and so encourages water retention. It is encouraged by drinking tea, coffee and alcohol, all of which are not only strong diuretics, but also make you excrete precious minerals like magnesium and potassium, which help to prevent water retention.

Your body doesn't need tea, coffee and alcohol. What

your body needs is water. Water not only hydrates you, it helps to flush out the wastes and toxins that make your body hold on to water in order to dilute them. Imagine washing your face in coffee or cola. If you wouldn't use these to clean your face with, how can they help to clean you inside? We all need to drink at least 4-8 glasses of water a day—more if you are very active.

Drinking less water will not cure water retention and could make it worse.

Water retention cause number 6
Lack of exercise

As we saw in the stories from people who suddenly gained water weight after a long flight or even from sitting still for hours in a meeting room, water retention can develop if you don't get enough exercise. This is because exercise is needed to stimulate your lymphatic system – an 'overflow' system which helps to drain your tissues. A lack of exercise results in lymphatic congestion, which causes water retention. 'Couch potatoes', beware!

Summary

Now that you know more about the causes of water retention, you will realize that a diet to lose water retention is not the same as a diet to lose fat, even if your ultimate aim is to get a lower reading on your weighing scales. Losing water retention is not about low-calorie eating and appetite control. The water retention diet (Waterfall Diet) is a *medical* diet which targets the main causes of Type II water retention, and helps your tissues release accumulated fluid and your kidneys (assuming they are normal and healthy) turn it into urine which you can excrete.

CHAPTER SIX
THE EASY WATER RETENTION DIET

I will tell you straight away that the original Waterfall Diet instructions work best, but a lot of people never get round to actually following them. They can seem a little complicated, and they also require a full six weeks of abstinence from anything made from

- Wheat (bread, flour, cakes, biscuits, cookies, sauces)
- Dairy products (milk, yoghurt, cheese, cream, butter)
- Eggs (desserts,
- Convenience foods
- Red meat
- Tea, coffee, salt, sugar (including chocolate, sweets and candies), artificial sweeteners and food additives

The original Waterfall Diet also asks you to be a home cook, using fresh, natural ingredients consisting of fruit, vegetables, fish, nuts, gluten-free grains, olive oil, herbs and spices.

Since many people in the western world now live on convenience foods and hardly cook at all, it is not surprising that those who are used to less strict forms of dieting may find it hard to get started. Since the Waterfall Diet is a medical diet, it does need to be strictly adhered to, otherwise it simply won't work. But the good news is that the first part is only a *test*, to help you find out which foods are safe for you to eat. As described in Georgie's case report, several pounds of retained water can be lost extremely quickly during this test, so it is well worth doing it properly.

So what's the difference between the *Easy Water Retention Diet* and the original *Waterfall Diet*?

The answer is that I've made the test phase of the diet less complicated and much shorter—only one week. During this week, you will be avoiding foods that most often trigger water retention in susceptible people. By avoiding these foods or ingredients, you have a 70 per cent chance of losing 2 to 10 lbs of retained water during this week. I hope you'll agree that these odds are well worth following a strict diet just for one week.

What happens after a week?

The good news is that after a week the test is over and if you have lost your water retention we only have to identify

EASY WATER RETENTION DIET

the exact problem foods. If you haven't lost any water weight, you no longer need to avoid any foods completely. You only need to concentrate on improving your everyday diet so that you can make better hormones and correct any weaknesses in your smallest blood vessels. It takes time for your body to make these repairs, but you should hopefully start to see results within two to three months.

CHAPTER SEVEN
SHOPPING AND COOKING

Apologies in advance if you don't think this diet looks very 'easy'. But you only have to do it for one week. It is a test to find out if your water retention can be released by avoiding some common ingredients. Unfortunately these ingredients are probably in most of your favourite foods! The test is also combined with a mild 'detox' which we find helps to kick-start the water release process.

During this week, please don't cheat. If you do, you must start the week again. This is a test, and if it's not done properly you will be none the wiser as to what is causing your water retention.

Preparations

Please do your shopping in advance. You will need:

- Fresh or frozen fish and/or seafood. Any kind you like except tuna. Ocean fish is best. (Tuna is not recommended as it contains small amounts of toxic mercury, which is very bad for your kidneys.) If you really cannot eat any form of fish

EASY WATER RETENTION DIET

you will have to make do with chicken or other white meat, but try to find some good quality free range chicken.

- Fresh or frozen vegetables: any kind—carrots, onions, greens, broccoli, cauliflower, cabbage or a mixture. Just stock up on a week's supply of whichever ones you like best and make sure that if it's a packet it contains just pure vegetables and nothing else.
- Fresh salad vegetables: tomatoes, peppers, celery, spring onions (scallions), radishes, rocket (arugula), parsley, avocados.
- Fresh or frozen fruit: those that fight water retention are oranges (especially the white pith and peel), and purple fruit like blueberries, blackberries, black cherries and black grapes.
- Dried beans or lentils if you are a good cook and know how to prepare them. Otherwise plain beans or lentils canned in plain water with no sugar or salt. You may need to buy them online or from a health food store.
- Olive oil.
- Potatoes and rice (preferably brown rice)
- Gluten free breakfast cereal. Look in health food stores or in the 'free from' section of the supermarket, or buy online.
- Non-dairy milk for cereals and smoothies. Most people use soy milk*. Health food stores also sell milk made from rice or almonds. *If you have read any criticisms of soy, please consider reading

Appendix III. If you think you may be allergic to soy, please do not consume it.
- Nuts: Brazils, cashews, pecans, almonds, walnuts, macadamias, peanuts etc. Brazils are best, but buy whatever you like best, unsalted.
- Garlic, chilli, ginger, either fresh or powdered.
- Herbal tea: cinnamon spice tea/bags, green tea/bags.

Optional extras: fresh fruit juice (no sugar, sweeteners or additives), quinoa, millet, buckwheat, canned tomatoes or passata (no salt or additives), salmon, herring or sardines canned in oil or plain water, cocoa powder, coconut milk, coconut cream, sunflower oil or other types of nut or seed oil, black pepper, fresh or dried herbs or spices, mushrooms, plain unflavoured tofu, ginger and lemon tea/bags, sheep or goat milk yoghurt, preservative-free dried fruit, gelatine, sodium-free salt substitute, sparkling mineral water (good for mixing with fresh fruit juice).

You do not have to buy anything you really don't like or don't want to cook, but please ensure you end up with a good variety. If you can't find these ingredients locally, you can buy them online from Amazon.com or other websites. Vegetarians can leave out the meat and fish, and eat more beans, lentils, rice, tofu and nuts instead.

Use these ingredients to make your own simple meals for one week. You will find some recipes in Appendix II. You can make any of the combinations suggested below. As long as you only use the ingredients listed here you can also make up your own combinations. This is not a calorie-controlled diet, so as regards portion sizes you must use

EASY WATER RETENTION DIET

your own judgment and common sense. The only rule is that for one whole week nothing at all except plain water and the foods and drinks listed here should pass your lips. Absolutely no food additives such as sweeteners or preservatives are allowed, so either avoid convenience foods completely, or check all labels carefully. If you make a mistake, even if you consume only tiny, trace amounts of foods that are not on this list, you must start again. This is not a conventional type of diet, it is a test requiring strictly controlled conditions.

Breakfast suggestions

- Gluten free cereal with non-dairy milk, bananas and chopped almonds.
- Fish poached gently in water and served with grilled (broiled) tomatoes plus mushrooms pan-fried with olive oil and chopped parsley
- Avocado smoothie: whizz an avocado with non-dairy milk, a handful of strawberries and a tablespoon of ground almonds (almond flour)

Lunches and Suppers

- Cooked brown rice or buckwheat tossed with olive oil and lemon juice, chopped parsley, celery and radish, and grated carrot
- Chopped cucumber and mint mixed with sheep or goat yoghurt (makes a good topping for rice salads, baked potato or canned fish)

- Poached or canned salmon, herrings or sardines (canned in plain unsalted water or oil)
- Hot lentil soup made with lentils, onion, garlic, ginger, chilli, parsley and olive oil
- Hot celery, watercress and potato soup
- Cooked beans or chickpeas (garbanzo beans) with olive oil and lemon juice, chopped celery, parsley and spring onion (scallion)
- Warm salad of roasted peppers, tomatoes and courgettes (zucchini) with olive oil, lemon juice and grated orange or lemon zest
- Avocado with prawns (shrimps) and rocket (arugula) with olive oil and lemon juice.

Main Meals

- Pan-fried fish which has been coated with ground herbs, spices and pepper before frying. Served with baked potato or roasted vegetables
- Stir-fry of rice noodles, tofu and frozen mixed vegetables
- Casserole of beans or chicken with onions, broccoli, carrots and tomato
- Baked potato topped with sheep or goat yoghurt mixed with chopped spring onion (scallion) and garlic
- Lentil or bean burgers or tofu burgers with green salad and grated radish
- Cooked brown rice, millet or buckwheat baked with finely chopped onion, carrot, celery and

cabbage and topped with soya (soy) yoghurt or sheep's yoghurt.
- Thai curries with vegetables, prawns (shrimps) or tofu, coconut milk and rice noodles

Desserts

Many fruits can be stewed: placed in a lidded casserole dish with a tablespoon of water and heated in a moderate oven until the juices run. Try this with blueberries, plums, raspberries and chopped apple or mango. Stir in preservative-free dried fruit for added sweetness, or chopped nuts, and serve with coconut milk or sheep or goat yoghurt, or warm rice pudding made with non-dairy milk. Adding gelatine to hot fruit and fruit juice makes delicious jelly desserts once cooled. Good fruits to eat fresh include peaches, bananas, melons and strawberries.

Snacks

Fresh or roasted nuts and peanuts (without salt) are a filling snack, but can pile on the calories relatively quickly, so eat them with a hot drink or some fresh fruit to help you feel fuller.

Fresh fruit can make a good snack, but don't eat it on its own if it leaves you feeling hungry sooner. Save it for dessert after meals, or eat it together with other snacks e.g. a slice of cold chicken, a bowl of hot lentil soup, gluten-free cereal or left-over rice salad.

Drinks

Fruit juices should be diluted half and half with water. Fresh natural fruit juice (with a little citrus zest whizzed in) is actually quite delicious mixed with sparkling mineral water, and is much better than artificial canned sodas.

Try to drink green tea and cinnamon spice tea as often as you can. These contain ingredients which help to warm up your metabolism and control your blood sugar levels.

Drinking plain water absorbs wastes and toxins and helps to carry them out of the body.

Side effects to look out for

It's best to start this diet on a Friday since most people feel a bit tired on the second and third days (a good sign), and the lack of caffeine may make you develop a headache. Take a plain aspirin if you need to, the cheapest one you can find, which means it contains the least number of additives. Please don't take other types of painkillers, especially paracetamol/acetaminofen, which is toxic. If you feel unwell, just rest and concentrate on the benefits.

If you are not used to eating vegetables you may also get some intestinal gas, which can be reduced with double-strength cinnamon spice tea and by using ginger and chilli in cooking.

Can I eat...?

Please don't get in a tangle with 'can I eat?' questions or you will never get started with the diet. One of my readers wanted to know if she could continue consuming 'wheat grass'. If you have to ask then just assume the answer is 'no', and get on with the test!

What happens next?

If you haven't noticed any water retention loss during the test week, please skip to the next section. On the other hand, if you have been urinating a lot more than usual, and seem to be retaining less water, the next step is to find out which are your problem foods. We know that you have problem foods, because otherwise you would not have lost water retention so quickly. Rapid water retention loss on this diet always means that you have stopped consuming something that was upsetting your normal water balance.

Potential problem foods

Most people's problem foods are:
- Salt, as found in almost all convenience foods, stock (broth) cubes, smoked and processed meats, and even bread.
- Wheat and other gluten-containing grains, as found in bread, rye bread, oats, biscuits (cookies), cakes, pastries, pasta, flour, sauces, and crispy coatings on fried foods.
- Cows milk products, as found in milk, cheese, yoghurt, butter, cream, ice cream, and in small amounts in many commercial convenience foods.
- Yeast, as found in bread and alcoholic drinks

- Egg, which is used in small amounts in a very wide variety of commercial foods including ice cream, pastries and cakes.
- Corn (maize).
- Soy can also be a problem food for a few people.

To find out your problem food(s)

You will need to stay on the basic test diet a little longer while you add one food at a time from the potential problem food list above. It is extremely likely that you won't find this too difficult if you are feeling much better, as most people are at this stage. Starting with salt, add one food at a time back into your diet to see whether it brings any pains, drowsiness, stuffy nose, rashes or water weight. Eat it every day for five days. If you get any symptoms, stop eating it and wait until you feel better before moving on to the next food. If it does not seem to be a problem food, you can continue to eat it.

Some of you will discover that the problem food is salt, for others it will be gluten-containing grains, and for others, dairy products. Some people are also sensitive to corn, yeast, soy or egg, but these are by no means such common water retention triggers as the first three foods. Almost anything can become a problem food at some point in your life, even if you never had a problem with it before. If you'd like to learn more about this, I recommend reading my book The Waterfall Diet, which has more detailed explanations.

What to do when your test is complete

If any food tested positive, continue to avoid it for at least six months. You may then be able to tolerate a little of this food from time to time without a return of your water retention.

If the test diet really helped you, but you could not identify a particular food, then you may be sensitive to something that was not tested. The best way to find out is to keep a food diary. Write down when your symptoms occurred, and what you had recently eaten. The idea is to narrow down the possible culprits.

If you did not feel any different after a week on the test diet, go to the next section: improving your eating habits.

Improving your eating habits

Whatever the result of the one-week test, it is important to understand that the average western diet as eaten in the English-speaking countries and Europe (and increasingly in urban areas in the rest of the world) may not seem to cause any problems while you are young, but as you get older, your hormones and immune system, nervous system, energy, bones, and ability to detoxify your body, can start to weaken. Your DNA and genes determine how well your body can cope with your eating habits, and which parts of your body are weaker than others, but ultimately if we have any symptoms like skin problems, water retention, insomnia, nervous problems or feeling easily tired, it is a sign that our eating habits need to change. In the next chapter you will find my Guide to Healthy Living.

CHAPTER EIGHT
GUIDE TO HEALTHY LIVING

'You are what you eat' is something we hear over and over again. But official advice can be confusing. Health advice comes from so many sources, and it's all different. But don't let that frustrate you. Sometimes we misinterpret what we read and assume the worst. In fact, for good health you don't need to avoid every scrap of salt, fat, chocolate or fried food. The secret is learning how to balance treats with healthy foods so that they don't stress your metabolism.

Health Tip 1: Reduce Sugar

The number one enemy to saying slim and healthy is sugar. Everything that is sweetened needs to be rationed. Aim to eat or drink no more than one sweetened item a day. If you can't bear tea or coffee without sugar, then just have one cup of tea or coffee a day.

Sugar has a double-whammy effect on your weight. Its calories are turned into fat, and as you get older it makes your body produce more of a hormone that stops you losing weight when you diet.

This hormone (called insulin) is the reason why many people in their forties start to put on weight around their middle no matter how little they eat. Known as the 'apple shape', this is very hard to control and is linked with heart disease and diabetes. Insulin also promotes water retention by making you retain sodium.

Artificial Sweeteners?

Recent research shows that artificial sweeteners make your body produce just as much insulin as sugary items. Research also shows that sweeteners increase hunger and make you eat more. So-called 'diet' foods and drinks often contain artificial sweeteners, so don't rely on them to keep you slim.

Health Tip 2: More Veg Less Meat

Research shows that any more than about four ounces (110 grams) of animal protein a day starts to make us accumulate acids and ammonia and is not very healthy, especially for our kidneys—the key organ for water excretion.

The World Health Organization warns that eating red meat more than twice a week (especially if charred by barbecuing etc) substantially increases our risk of cancer.

On the other hand fresh fruit and vegetables (preferably five portions a day) help to prevent many diseases. Women especially need to eat broccoli, cabbage and cauliflower several times a week, as these are incredibly protective against breast cancer and can help you eliminate toxins that might encourage water retention.

Instead of eating mostly salads and fruits when you diet, try eating chunky vegetable and bean soup. It's tasty and satisfying! See some of my healthy recipes in Appendix II.

Health Tip 3: Less Alcohol

Alcohol is toxic to every single cell in your body, especially your liver. It is a major cause of several cancers, and should be reserved for special occasions only. Alcohol can make you more prone to water retention by dehydrating you.

Health Tip 4: Less Pastry And White Flour, More Whole-Grain Foods

Try learning how to make your own pastry crusts, cakes, biscuits and cookies so that you can see how much fat goes into them. You will be shocked. There is very little nutritional value in these foods, just calories. White bread and pasta is little better. On the other hand whole-grain foods help to protect you from B-vitamin and magnesium deficiencies that harm your water balance, nervous system, glands and metabolism.

Health Tip 5: Less Deep-Fried Food

Deep-fried foods such as potato chips, fries, crisps, crispy snacks and items fried in batter or breadcrumbs absorb large amounts of fat. When heated and re-used for cooking, fats and oils develop toxins which increase your risk of cancer. Try not to eat these foods more than once a week or so, or they could encourage vitamin and mineral deficiencies.

Health Tip 6: Don't Smoke!

It makes you smelly, it give you dental abscesses and gum disease, it makes your teeth fall out, it ages you quickly, wrinkles and dries your skin, and damages your lungs. Any toxic habit like this can also encourage metabolic imbalances in your body. Need I say more?

Health Tip 7: Exercise Doesn't Have To Be A Bore

Exercise helps to protect you from the harmful effects of producing too much insulin. So if you find yourself retaining water and beginning to turn into an apple shape, you are definitely not getting enough exercise. Aim to get out of breath for at least 15 minutes, five days a week.

Working exercise into your daily routine helps to prevent it becoming a bore. Park your car at the top of a steep hill when you go to work or go shopping. Use stairs instead of lifts, escalators and elevators. Spend more time walking (especially fast walking) or cycling instead of driving.

CHAPTER NINE
SPECIAL ANTI-WATER RETENTION FOODS

Blueberries, bilberries and other blue and purple fruits

These fruits are the richest source of flavonoids, which help to keep your smallest blood vessels—your capillaries—strong. Without enough flavonoids in your diet, capillaries get weak and leaky and this encourages water retention, especially in the legs, feet and ankles.

Some herbal products are actually consumed because of their flavonoid content. For instance the flavonoid content of the product Ginkgo biloba is the reason for its beneficial effect on the smallest blood vessels in the brain. Orange and lemon zest (including the white part) are another good source of flavonoids.

Celery, celery juice and parsley

These are the richest sources of coumarin, a natural substance which is also found in grass and helps to give milk its rich flavour. Coumarin stimulates the immune system to break down waste particles which have become trapped in the tissues and lie there attracting excess fluid.

These foods are very useful in combating water retention. It is possible to buy celery juice in some larger health food stores, but far cheaper to buy an inexpensive juice extractor machine and some bunches of celery, and make the juice yourself. You will need to drink 1-2 medium-sized wineglasses a day (or the equivalent), so it's a good idea to get well stocked up. Your celery juice can be kept in the fridge for a few days, or you could freeze it or make it into soup. Whizz in a handful of parsley to make it even more effective. You can add tomato, apple or lemon juice to the celery for extra flavour, or even chilli or ginger, but no salt.

An added bonus is that celery juice and parsley also have a mild diuretic action, so they can both draw fluid out of your tissues and help your kidneys turn it into urine. Very useful foods indeed!

Almonds, sunflower and sesame seeds

Together with oats, oatmeal and leafy green vegetables, these are some of the best sources of magnesium, a mineral which is often lacking in the western diet but plays a vital role in the body's water balance. These food items also provide vitamin B6 and zinc, which perform many tasks together with magnesium.

Broccoli, brussels sprouts, cauliflower, cabbage and kale

These are not only rich in magnesium, they also help a woman's body to break down excessively high oestrogen (estrogen) levels which can encourage not just water retention, but PMS, fibroids, ovarian cysts and endometriosis.

Avocados

Avocados are one of the richest sources of vitamin B6. This vitamin is intimately involved in the production of hormones which help to control water balance, and it also aids the absorption of magnesium.

Warm food and warming spices

Unless you live in a very warm part of the world, or unless you are a very hot-blooded athletic person, you may find that dieting on cold food and raw salads just intensifies your cravings for 'comfort food'. In oriental medicine cold and raw foods would be considered to encourage weight gain as they depletes the body's 'fire' or Yang energy. You will find hot lentil soup, and casseroles flavoured with garlic, onion, chives, cayenne, chilli and ginger much more energizing. Oriental experts believe that such foods actually burn off excess water in our bodies, and this is very good news for water retention sufferers.

Don't overdo the spices—burning your insides would be counter-productive and unnecessary. Another tip (if you can stand it!) do try to take a quick cold shower every morning. This really stimulates your metabolism!

If any of the foods mentioned in this book are new to you, try consulting the staff at your local health food store. They will usually be delighted to help you find items such as celery juice and sunflower seeds, or to tell you how to make your own juices using a juice extractor machine.

APPENDIX I
HERBAL AND NUTRITIONAL SUPPLEMENTS

Herbal diuretics such as dandelion leaf and boldo work in a similar way to prescription diuretics—they artificially stimulate your kidneys to drain fluid out of your blood. This means that they are really only suitable for Type I water retention. They are not used in the natural treatment of Type II water retention because they could aggravate the problem, just like prescription diuretics.

But some herbal medicines don't work by artificially stimulating your kidneys. They work by enhancing the therapeutic effects of the water retention diet, for instance by helping to strengthen the walls of the smallest blood vessels, helping to decongest the lymphatic system, helping the liver get rid of toxins, and helping the immune system break down waste particles which have become trapped in the tissues and lie there attracting water. Below is a list of the recommended herbal medicines:

- Red clover
- Ginkgo biloba
- Horse chestnut
- Silymarin (an extract of the herb milk thistle)
- Gotu kola
- Butcher's broom
- Cornsilk (can be used for swollen legs in the last 3 months of pregnancy)

Nutritional supplements cannot take the place of healthy eating, but if you are committed to make the change to a healthier lifestyle they can speed up your body's ability to repair its metabolism. A list of recommended herbal and nutritional supplements can be found here:

For readers in UK / Europe

www.health-diets.net/links/linda-recommends-uk/

For readers in the USA and rest of world

www.health-diets.net/links/linda-recommends/

APPENDIX II
RECIPES

How to cook lentils

A quantity of lentils can be prepared in advance and will keep in the fridge for up to 4 days, or can be frozen. They are rich in protein, B vitamins and iron.

Use half a cup / 115 ml uncooked lentils per serving. Put the lentils in a large pan and add about 2½ times their volume of boiling water plus a tablespoon of olive oil to stop them frothing up too much. Never add salt at this stage, as it will toughen them. Bring to the boil and simmer for 25-40 minutes, depending on the size and age of the lentils. Stir occasionally. Red lentils take only 25 minutes. Brown, green or yellow lentils take 30 to 40 minutes. Lentils boil over easily, which is why it is a good idea to use a pan several sizes larger than you would normally need.

To freeze cooked lentils, allow them to cool and put spoonfuls in the wells of tart or muffin baking tins. Freeze the tins then empty out the frozen lentils, put them in bags and return to the freezer.

How to cook brown rice

Brown rice is much more nutritious than white. It is available from supermarkets and health food stores. You can cook brown rice using the directions on the packet, but this method is my favourite. Use half a cup / 115 ml rice per serving. Pre-soak the rice overnight in at least twice its volume of cold water. Before cooking, drain the rice, add enough boiling water to cover it, bring to the boil then cover the pan tightly with a lid and simmer on the lowest possible heat until tender (about 25 minutes). By now the water should all have been absorbed. If not, drain the rice in a sieve and replace it immediately in the pan. Replace the lid and leave the rice in the covered pan away from the heat for five minutes, after which it is ready to serve.

Once cold, brown rice can be spread out on an oiled baking tray, frozen, then crumbled into grains and bagged for the freezer.

How to stew fruit

Berries are ideal for stewing. Fresh berries are best, but frozen are usually a cheaper option.

EASY WATER RETENTION DIET

Use a cupful of berries for each serving. Place in a small pan with 2 tbsp water, over a gentle heat. Put the lid on the pan and leave it, checking and shaking the pan from time to time. When the berries are warm and juice is running from them, they are ready. Serve warm or cold, with coconut milk.

Sample recipes

These can be adapted, using other ingredients in your shopping list.

Breakfast smoothie

For each serving
> 1 cup / 235 ml soy milk
> half an avocado
> 1 level tbsp ground almonds (almond flour)
> 1 handful fresh or frozen berries

Whizz in a blender until smooth. Drink immediately otherwise the avocado may spoil.

Salad of roasted peppers, tomatoes and courgettes (zucchini)

For each serving
> 1 red or green (bell) pepper, deseeded and quartered
> 2 tomatoes, halved
> 1 medium courgette (zucchini), cut lengthwise in half and then into 2-inch segments
> 4 tbsp olive oil

1 tbsp lemon juice

A thumb-sized piece of orange or lemon peel, finely shredded with a sharp knife

Preheat oven to 400F/200C/Gas 6. Put the vegetable pieces and shredded peel on an oiled baking tray, brush with 2 tbsp olive oil, and place the baking tray in the oven for 30 minutes or until the vegetables are tender and beginning to brown.

When cooked, remove from the oven, allow to cool, then toss in a bowl with the lemon juice and the remaining olive oil. Season with salt substitute and freshly ground black pepper.

Green lentil soup with white fish, cabbage, ginger and chives

For each serving

1 cup / 235 ml cooked green lentils

4 oz / 115 grams white fish, filleted and cut into bite-sized chunks

1 handful green cabbage, finely shredded

1 thumb-sized piece of fresh ginger, finely chopped

1 tbsp lemon juice

1 tsp chives, chopped

Boiling water

See the beginning of this section for how to cook lentils. Put the cooked lentils in a saucepan and stir in enough boiling water to produce a soupy but not watery consistency. Stir in the shredded cabbage and ginger and bring to the boil over a medium heat. Simmer gently for five minutes, stirring occasionally, then season with salt substitute and add the chives and fish pieces. Return the pan to the heat, bring back to boiling point and immediately remove from the heat. Cover the pan and leave for two minutes. Check that the fish is cooked through (check to see that it flakes easily) and serve.

Thai chicken or tofu curry

For each serving
>   1 raw chicken breast, cut into thin strips
>   Or 110 g / 4 oz tofu cut into bite-size chunks
>   1/2 cup / 115 ml mixed chopped frozen vegetables (e.g. corn kernels, peppers, carrots)
>   Generous 3/4 cup or 200 ml canned coconut milk
>   60 g / 2 oz fine dried rice noodles or vermicelli
>   2 tbsp groundnut or olive oil
>   1 tsp red Thai curry paste

Heat the oil in a stir-fry pan over a medium heat, add the chicken strips or tofu chunks and stir-fry until golden. Remove from the pan and put to one side. Add the curry paste to the same pan, stir briefly then pour in the coconut milk, followed by the chopped vegetables and the cooked chicken. Bring to the boil and simmer gently, stirring, until the vegetables are tender and the chicken cooked through. Meanwhile put the rice noodles in a bowl and cover with boiling water to soften for a few minutes. Drain thoroughly in a sieve, place in a serving dish and stir in the rice milk, chicken and vegetables. Season with salt substitute and serve.

APPENDIX III
SOY FACTS

When my first book on water retention, the *Waterfall Diet* was first published, people in the UK gave it a very high rating, but I was surprised to see that, according to some readers' comments on Amazon.com, people in the US had mixed reactions. The book contains some recipes based on tofu and suggests soy milk as a substitute for cow's milk, which is not allowed in the first few weeks of the waterfall diet. I was amazed to see that there are people in the US who view soy foods almost like a poison. This view is virtually unheard of in the UK.

This apparently strange attitude to soy seems to come from a campaign which a small group of people have been conducting for about 20 years. It all started with a very unfortunate story about bird breeders in New Zealand whose baby birds developed abnormalities after being given a new feed based on soy. Concerns about feeding large amounts of concentrated, processed soy to young animals and human babies are clearly valid. However there should not be any problem with a moderate intake of traditional soy foods for adults. People in China and Japan have been consuming these foods for hundreds—if not thousands of years, and consider them to be a valuable part of their diet.

On the other hand highly concentrated soy products, such as soy protein isolate, soy isoflavone supplements and imitation meat products made from soy, have indeed been linked with detrimental effects to the thyroid gland. In my view these foods should be avoided as they are far too concentrated.

The feelings of the anti-soy campaigners are understandable, but though well-meant, their persistent warnings about all forms of soy could be inappropriate, especially when they say that soy causes breast cancer. What they claim is: soy contains plant oestrogens (estrogens). Most cases of breast cancer are caused by excessive oestrogen. Therefore if you don't want to get breast cancer, you had better avoid soy.

But as pointed out many times by experts such as biochemist Dr Jeffrey Bland, soy isoflavones (the active ingredients) are not oestrogens but oestrogen modulators or balancers. This means they have binding proteins which can latch on to excessive oestrogen in a woman's body and block it from doing harm. If there is not enough oestrogen around, they also have a weakly oestrogenic effect which can help to make good the deficit.

Now an amazing new study on 5,000 women with

breast cancer has emerged from China, where 20% or more of the dietary protein comes from soy. It seems that the women with the highest soy intake had the lowest risk of cancer death or recurrence, and the women with the lowest soy intake had the highest risk.

Many pollutants such as PCBs exert their harmful effects by acting as artificial oestrogens in the body, so I for one will continue to eat my daily pot of fruit-flavoured soy yoghurt!

GM soy

Some readers have also expressed concern that much of today's soy is genetically modified. This is a legitimate concern, but it can be addressed by checking out a company's policy on GM avoidance before buying its products. Certified organic soy products are the safest in this respect, as a product cannot legally be given organic certification unless it uses suppliers who ingredients test negative for GM content.

Soy allergy

Many people get strange reactions such as skin rashes or headaches after consuming common foods. Mostly these foods are wheat, gluten or dairy products, but some people also react to soy. Soy allergy is not very common in the UK, Europe and Australia, but may be more common in the United States.

RESOURCES

More recipes suitable for the water retention diet can be found in other books by Linda Lazarides, including the *Waterfall Diet*, the *Big Healthy Soup Diet* (in the U.S. this is titled as *Linda's Soup Diet Secrets*), and her forthcoming book the new edition of the *Gourmet Nutritional Therapy Cookbook*.

If you have a weight problem that includes the need for fat loss, *Linda's Flat Stomach Secrets* is a cutting-edge weight loss and body-shaping program packed with little-known facts that can help you avoid common mistakes and assumptions.

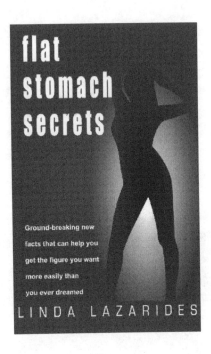

Have you ever wondered what causes middle-age spread? Why does the waistline keep expanding after a certain age, even if you are exercising the same and not eating any more?

Packed with little-known information, *Linda's Flat Stomach Secrets* explains the five causes of an expanding waistline and includes a comprehensive program and 7-day diet to begin to tackle it. You could lose as much as three inches from your waistline in three months. Discover

- How to avoid developing obsessive food cravings
- How to rebalance the hormones that control belly fat

EASY WATER RETENTION DIET

- A cool way of walking that powerfully works out your tummy muscles at the same time
- What is intestinal plaque and how it can cause bloating
- A deep-cleansing routine to tackle bloating, gas and water retention.

Linda Lazarides is known for revealing startling and astonishing facts that few people know about. This book is no exception. When Linda was writing it she was shocked to discover that common methods which people believe will help them lose weight can actually put their fat gain hormones into overdrive. This book is a 'must read' for anyone who is watching their waistline.

THE SCHOOL OF MODERN NATUROPATHY

Have you ever thought about training as a naturopathic nutritionist? This is a natural health consultant who specializes in creating tailored health programs which can help individuals overcome common health problems and ailments.

Linda Lazarides teaches a one-year diploma course by distance learning, using a combination of specially written course modules and internet-based teaching. This course is accredited by major organizations in the United Kingdom, United States, Australia and New Zealand. Graduates are also eligible to practice in Canada. Upon successful completion, you would be qualified to work as a wellness counsellor, health coach, naturopathic nutritionist or nutrition advisor. You would be eligible to set up in private practice, or work in a health club, health food store or perhaps for a vitamin or natural products company.

If you plan to work as a writer or journalist, you would gain an in-depth understanding of holistic health which would greatly improve the quality of your books and articles and also make it much easier for you to find ideas and reliable information for articles to interest your readers.

Linda Lazarides is a master practitioner and founder of the British Association for Nutritional Therapy. In 1996 she helped the University of Westminster to set up the UK's first degree course in Nutritional Therapy. and previously for several years worked as a complementary practitioner for the British National Health Service. She has been a nutrition editor for the *International Journal of Alternative and Complementary Medicine*, an advisor to several national organizations, and has been invited to speak at parliamentary committees in the UK.

For more information about the School of Modern Naturopathy, and to read the course prospectus, please visit www.naturostudy.org.

Made in the USA
San Bernardino, CA
02 November 2016